UNDERSTANDING FIBROMYALGIA:

A GUIDE FOR FAMILY AND FRIENDS

BETTY DOTTERER

PAUL DAVIDSON, M.D.

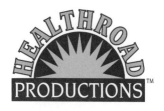

HEALTHROAD PRODUCTIONS
P.O. Box 2176
STATELINE, NEVADA 89449

Acknowledgements

We thank the thousands of people from whom we have learned about the real world of fibromyalgia. Many have taught us what helps, and others have taught us what makes it worse. All have contributed in one way or another to our understanding of fibromyalgia, how family and friends are affected and how they can offer support. Also, our thanks to Neva Beach for her insight and editorial suggestions.

Library of Congress Catalog Card Number: 96-77600

Betty Dotterer
Paul Davidson, M.D.
Understanding Fibromyalgia: A Guide for Family and Friends

ISBN: 0-9653493-0-6

HealthRoad Productions
P.O. Box 2176
Stateline, Nevada 89449.

Designed by Scott Silverman

Printed in the United States of America

CONTENTS

INTRODUCTION

"My doctor says my muscle pains are caused by fibromyalgia." Hearing this from a family member or friend might seem, at first, like wonderful news, the light at the end of a long, hard search. At last there's a name for the mysterious condition that has invaded your lives – and now that it's named it can be tamed. Can't it?

Yes and no.

Fibromyalgia can be "tamed;" can be treated and eased and, sometimes, even diminished until the pains disappear or are so mild they're easily borne. But between naming and taming this disruptive condition, both you and the fibromyalgia patient must learn everything possible about it, and develop coping strategies that can restore the quality of your lives.

We've written this booklet to give you basic information about fibromyalgia and answer some of the most pressing questions that you, as a member of the patient's family or support system, are faced with. What you will read is not a theoretical treatise, but a practical discussion of the real world of fibromyalgia, based on what we've learned through many thousands of contacts with patients, from extensive interviews of patients and their families and friends, from support groups, medical literature, discussions with other physicians and healthcare professionals, and dealings with insurance companies and disability carriers.

The key to controlling fibromyalgia is knowledge. Reading this booklet will set you on the path to understanding this condition and show you how to be a positive participant in your friend or family member's recovery.

HELPING THE FIBROMYALGIA PATIENT

If someone in your family or a friend has fibromyalgia, you've probably said or thought at least some of these things:

- I've never heard of fibromyalgia. What is it?
- But you don't look sick.
- What did your doctor say?
- How can all your tests be normal when you feel so ill?
- Are you sure the doctor understands your problems?
- I wonder why the medication isn't helping?
- Maybe you just need more exercise.
- Maybe it's all in your head.
- It says here that you'll be in pain for the rest of your life! Is that true?
- I really want to help you, but what can I *do*?

It can be tremendously frustrating when you want to help but don't know how. And it can be maddeningly difficult to find helpful information about fibromyalgia, or FMS as it's often called. But it's crucially important for you, as family member or friend, to get at least some elementary understanding of this little-known but very real condition. If you don't, you may not only be of no help, but your frustrations may lead you to unwittingly contribute to the FMS patient's illness.

This booklet will give you the information and guidance needed by everyone who has an FMS patient in his/her life. You can read about this condition in more detail in Dr. Davidson's book, *Chronic Muscle Pain Syndrome*[1], and other resources listed in the back, but here you will find the essential information – and more about what FMS means to you, as a part of the FMS patient's support system. We will give you practical information and insight into the world of FMS, show you what has been learned about the syndrome, and offer a variety of things you can do to help your FMS family member or friend and yourself.

Before going any further, keep in mind these two basic facts:

The pain of FMS is real.
FMS is a treatable condition.

WHAT IS FMS?

Fibromyalgia is considered a syndrome, that is, a number of symptoms that occur together and characterize a specific condition. In 1990, the American College of Rheumatology (ACR) presented two criteria for diagnosing FMS:[2]

- Widespread muscle pain of at least three months duration in combination with
- Tenderness at 11 or more of the 18 specific tender point sites. ("Tender point sites" aren't sore places on the body. Rather, they are specific places that hurt when measured pressure is applied.)

One of the hallmarks of FMS is the lack of objective findings in patients. The methods doctors routinely use to diagnose and understand disease–X-rays, biopsies, MRI tests, bone scans, blood tests and so on–show no abnormal results in patients with FMS. The tender points criteria, above, is the only consistent physical finding when testing for this condition.

While there are only two symptoms included in the official ACR criteria for FMS, many other symptoms are often present in a higher percentage of FMS patients than in the general population. Here is a brief recap of the most common ones–you are sure to recognize at least some of them in your family member or friend's case:

- <u>Chronic muscle aches, pains, and stiffness</u>. The important word here is chronic.
- <u>Fatigue</u>. FMS patients may wake up in the morning feeling as tired as when they went to bed. They may complain that they feel listless, have no energy for work or pleasure.

- <u>Sleep disorders</u>. People with FMS often report difficulty in getting to sleep, or restless sleep, often accompanied by muscle aches and pains in the night.
- <u>Headaches</u>. Both tension and migraine headaches may accompany FMS.
- <u>Irritable bowel syndrome</u>. FMS patients may complain of both constipation and loose bowel movements, as well as gas, distention, and abdominal cramping.
- <u>Pain in the upper jaw when chewing or opening the mouth</u>. This is known as temporomandibular joint syndrome or TMJ syndrome.
- <u>Feelings of joint pain and swelling</u>. About half of people with FMS have pain in their joints and a sense that the joints are swollen, when no swelling is actually present.
- <u>Feelings of numbness or tingling in the extremities</u>. These feelings are common in FMS, however they are not due to abnormal nerve damage or function.
- <u>Anxiety or depression</u>. These are very common among FMS patients, and we will have more to say about them later.

All these symptoms are real, and can have serious effects on both the patient's life and your own. But it is also important to know some things that FMS does not do:

FMS does not cause deformity.
FMS does not lead to arthritis.
FMS does not shorten life-expectancy.

ABOUT FMS

FMS has been known through medical literature for over 150 years. It most certainly existed long before that–perhaps as long as humans have walked on the earth–but until relatively recently there has been little understanding of the condition or how to treat it.

The symptoms that are now called fibromyalgia were first

described in 1843 by Dr. Robert Froriep, a German physician[3], and it was in German and Scandinavian medical literature that mention of muscle pain symptoms were found, for the rest of the 19th century. The symptoms were thought to result from abnormalities within the muscles, which could be corrected by medication and purely physical means such as heat and massage and, later, by electrical stimulation.

In 1904 an English physician, Dr. William Gowers, gave the name fibrositis to the condition[4]. He assumed there was inflammation of the fibrous tissue, however no evidence of inflammation has ever been found. Modest medical research continued until around the onset of WW II, but with no success. No one was able to find anything wrong with the muscles or in any other part of the body. Frustrated researchers turned their attention to other, fields such as infectious diseases, heart disease, arthritis, cancer and the like.

Then, in the early 1980s, first in Japan and Australia and soon in many other countries, industrial health experts became aware of a disturbing phenomenon. Although workers had complained of muscle aches and pains for centuries, such complaints were starting to reach epidemic proportions. They were also becoming a huge financial burden on industry, since many of the workers were being cared for through various Workers Compensation insurance systems. Insurance premiums escalated to the point at which they sometimes threatened the very existence of many small companies. (FMS and health insurance is still a major issue, as we will see later.)

Since that time, FMS has come to be recognized as one of the major rheumatic conditions responsible for chronic muscle pain. An estimated six to twelve million Americans have FMS, ranging from mild to severe. When looked for, FMS has been found in every country in the world.

What causes FMS?

In researching and treating FMS the emphasis has now shifted away from the primarily mechanistic view. It has become obvious that FMS is not simply a biochemical derangement of bodily functions, nor is it purely psychological in origin, nor is it the body's response to environmental factors. As we mentioned earlier, in FMS, all laboratory tests and X-rays are normal. No single test or combination of tests clearly indicates why FMS occurs or gives accurate clues to its origin. It is a condition that results from the subtle – or often not-so-subtle – interactions of all three: body, mind, and environment. Although FMS can seemingly appear out of nowhere, one or more of the following factors often precede the onset of the illness:

- Restriction of physical activity such as illness or injury, or a job that is primarily sedentary.
- Physical deconditioning such as might result from lack of exercise or restriction of activities.
- Chronic muscle tension at home or on the job.
- Minor or major physical trauma, such as a minor sprain or a severe automobile accident.
- Infections of almost any kind: the flu, infectious mononucleosis, pneumonia, etc.
- Minor or major emotional trauma, such as:
  - Family, financial, or job stress.
  - Physical, sexual, or emotional abuse.
- Chronic illness such as rheumatoid arthritis, systemic lupus, or Sjögren's syndrome.

Approximately 90% of those affected with FMS are female. FMS most often has its onset between the ages of 20 and 50 years, however, it is known to affect children and those over 50 as well. There is increasing evidence that stressful events play major roles in the development of FMS. This raises another question: everyone has stress, so why do only some people suffer from this

7

condition? The answer here may lie in the susceptibility of the individual concerned–which leads to yet another question: why is one person susceptible and another not? To which there is currently no answer. We do not know.

Does FMS Go Away? Can It Be Cured?

The symptoms of FMS may improve spontaneously, by themselves. The greatest improvement, though, is in those patients who are able to recognize and cope with the many issues involved in causing FMS in the first place. For some people those issues are overwhelming, and there may be little or no improvement. In most, the causative problems can be dealt with and the patient's condition improved remarkably, to the point where the symptoms are very tolerable. In some, a complete disappearance of pain can be achieved.

So can FMS be cured? If a cure is understood to be a restoration to health, the answer is "Yes." If a cure is understood to mean "gone never to come back" the answer is "Possibly." But in any medical condition, if the causative factors all fall into place the condition will recur. So it is with FMS. And when improvement is made, that is the time to emphasize prevention.

Treating FMS

It has become clear that successful therapy requires that people with FMS must be deeply involved with their own therapy. They cannot rely *solely* on their physician or on anyone else. The healer within must work together with the healers without.

With all its technological marvels in some areas, modern medicine has not had a very good record in reducing or eliminating the pain of FMS until relatively recently. Modern ideas on the treatment of FMS emphasize a *multidisciplinary approach.* This means that the patient's body, mind, and environment must be examined to find the underlying factors that contribute to the muscle pain and other symptoms of FMS, then treated for each appropriately. Current approaches to therapy combine findings from several medical fields, such as, for example, those concerned with pain perception, pharmacology, exercise physiology, psychological stress, depression and anxiety. Intertwined with these are eastern concepts of the mind/body relationship. From all this a new and more effective approach has emerged.

Some elements of an effective modern therapy program for FMS are:

- Education
- Self-involvement and management; being proactive
- Physical conditioning
- A proper balance between exercise and rest
- Stress reduction
- Psychological support
- Treatment of anxiety and depression
- Cultivation of a hopeful, optimistic attitude
- Avoidance of disability
- The support and understanding of family and friends

The Role of Family and Friends

You are a crucial part of any FMS treatment program. Remember, healing takes place both inside the patient's body and mind, and outside, in his/her environment, both physical and human. The people around the FMS patient can make a major difference in the healing process. The difference you make can be negative–can make the FMS symptoms worse, or hinder the patient's own efforts at healing. Or it can be positive–can support the patient's efforts and be a major factor in bringing about reduction or even disappearance of FMS symptoms.

THE REAL WORLD OF FIBROMYALGIA: FEARS, FRUSTRATION AND FRIENDS

The person with FMS suffers not only from the pain of the condition itself. To that pain is often added the confusion and frustration of getting a correct diagnosis, finding a physician who is familiar with the condition and knows what treatments to recommend, accessing those treatments, and paying for them.

It's hard to walk in someone else's shoes, but it may help you understand what your friend or family member is going through if we follow an FMS patient through some typical real-life experiences.

Janet has chronic muscle pains and she knows that they are not simply in her mind. The pains are constant and widespread. She looks healthy, she has no deformities and a routine physical exam shows all of her laboratory tests as normal. Her pain persists, and she seeks more help.

From Her Physician

Janet's regular physician is one of those who, unfortunately, is unfamiliar with fibromyalgia, and has one or more of these reactions:

- We need more laboratory tests and X-rays.
- The tests are normal, so her pain doesn't exist.
- She's just trying to get disability.
- Every medicine I've tried doesn't work, and I'm frustrated.
- She may just need some physical therapy.
- I have no idea of what causes her pain. I'll refer her to Dr. S. for another opinion.

Janet, meanwhile, discovers the term FMS in her own research or from a friend who is familiar with the condition. She is enormously relieved to at least have a name for what's wrong with her, and has high hopes as she goes to her appointment with Dr. S., the physician she's been referred to. "I've got FMS," she says when giving her history. "That's 'fibromyalgia syndrome,'" she adds. Dr. S. at least does know the term, but, like many physicians, knows little about it and doubts the reality of the syndrome. His/her reaction might resemble one or more of these:

- It's all in her mind.
- FMS? There's no such thing. It's a "wastebasket" diagnosis.
- FMS exists, but Janet is overreacting.
- FMS exists, but I don't have the vaguest idea how to treat it.
- From what I've read, she'll be in pain for the rest of her life.
- I don't have time to research this to find out what's going on here.

Fortunately, Janet persists in her search for help and at last finds a physician who is sympathetic to her pain and has a thorough knowledge of the medical literature, as well as a considerable amount of experience in treating it. This time the physician's responses at least validate her pain, but may or may not lead to solutions:

- It is definitely fibromyalgia, and I am familiar with the problem.
- I know what kind of treatment program is needed, but we don't have that in our city.
- There is a treatment program, but unfortunately the medical insurance won't cover it.
- She's lucky – a program is available and she'll be able to get financial coverage.

Medical Insurance And Fibromyalgia

For too many FMS patients, the problem of financial coverage for treatment is added to their physical suffering and the difficulty of finding an informed physician.

The extent of medical insurance coverage for FMS varies considerably. Much depends on the terms of the policy, and, when the claim is reviewed, the adjuster's and medical consultant's knowledge of FMS. The increasing trend to managed care programs has generally resulted in a tendency towards less covered care in the case of FMS. A request for coverage from an insurance carrier may be met with responses such as:

- Fibro-what? Never heard of it.
- We do not recognize this condition as a valid diagnosis.
- Please ask your doctor to send us copies of your entire record, explain your condition, tell us why you need therapy, give us references to fibromyalgia, and we'll get back to you within 30 days.
- We will authorize two physical therapy visits, however your policy does not include biotherapy or psychology.
- We are familiar with fibromyalgia and your policy includes physical therapy, biotherapy and psychological support.

Medical Disability And FMS

Janet may apply for medical disability, through private insurance, Workers Compensation or Medicare. Again, a wide spectrum of responses may occur. Whether disability is granted depends upon a host of factors, some of which include the interpretation of physical and psychological symptoms, documented objective findings, the terms of the disability policy and how strictly they are enforced, the case manager's previous experiences with FMS, and the financial status and stability of the carrier. A reading of the literature from many countries shows us that disability is harder to come by when general economic conditions are not good. In the case of FMS, the inability to document any clear-cut physical findings compounds the problem.

Physical Therapists' Approaches To FMS

Let's return to Janet, who has been referred to a competent physical therapist. The therapist's training and experience, however, may or may not have offered exposure to and understanding of the condition of fibromyalgia. Here are a few scenarios of what Janet might find:

- She's treated solely with hot packs and massage and does not improve: some exercises are added, but Janet is worse after each session; stretching is added to the therapy program, but this does not help.
- Fibromyalgia is recognized, but the therapy program still doesn't help.
- The therapist recognizes fibromyalgia but is not sure of the best approach.
- The therapist recognizes fibromyalgia and works closely with Janet's physician to integrate physical therapy with a comprehensive treatment program.

Psychologists'/Psychiatrists' Approaches To FMS

Janet's physician, in desperation, refers her to a psychologist or psychiatrist, whose response could include opinions that:

- Janet has no problems that I can discern.
- Janet has anxiety and/or depression that preceded her pain.
- Janet has anxiety and/or depression because of her pain.
- I can see no relationship between her psychological situation and her pain.
- Janet has suffered trauma and abuse in her past, and these memories are interfering with her recovery.
- All pain has psychological aspects, and it is important to determine if these factors play a significant part in her pain.

If You Understand You Can Help!

As you've seen, the FMS patient carries a tremendous burden, not only of the very real pain of the condition, but of the confusion, ignorance, and resistance that is still common in the medical community and even more often in the insurance world. Your friend or family member may also have been exposed to a great deal of negative literature and talk, in the course of his/her search for information and help. Many writings about FMS are unduly pessimistic. They often state that the pain of fibromyalgia will be life-long and that permanent disability is the norm.

You can and must help counter this type of "doom and gloom" attitude. It can easily bring about a pessimistic state of mind–can even block the progress of treatment. A positive attitude is an asset when treating any chronic condition, and especially crucial with FMS. Fortunately, the facts about FMS more than justify optimism.

We have given you some glimpses of what FMS is all about, and what FMS patients, their family members and friends, may be experiencing. Your role in helping your family member or friend, based on your understanding, can be very positive. The next sections will focus on specific ways you can help.

THE IMPACT OF FMS ON RELATIONSHIPS

Having read this far, it should be obvious that a condition like this one can be very disruptive to the FMS patient's lifestyle and environment. This disruptive effect reverberates through the entire family and most other close relationships. How well these relationships endure the pressures and make the necessary adjustments is up to those of you who are involved.

You're taking the critical first step to success by reading this and learning more about FMS. Chances are you also understand the importance of the family's involvement when one member is in pain and struggling. Maybe you have a strong desire to help your loved one learn to manage FMS, or maybe you are just trying to restore some sort of order and control to your own life since FMS has become a part of it.

When someone is diagnosed with FMS they often feel vulnerable, lonely, and isolated. This can be a shock to family and friends, who may never have seen the FMS sufferer seem so dependent. A high percentage of FMS patients are exceptionally strong, self–sufficient people who may have never shown a vulnerable side in the past. Most people confronted with a painful medical condition will seek out close friends and family for comfort, but often the FMS patient's very strength takes friends and family by surprise. It can be hard to know how to respond to this sudden vulnerability. And if the FMS patient doesn't feel supported, he/she will begin to withdraw.

You may see your friend or loved one suffering physically as well as mentally. Self–esteem issues are common, as the FMS patient's energy and capabilities diminish. Many times the simplest tasks become very difficult or seemingly impossible. Tensions increase, as stresses build. Suddenly your friend or family member can feel too tired to go out to a movie, or attend an important school meeting. He/she may take disability leave from a previously rewarding job, and lose that important source of self-esteem. Tensions continue to mount, with spiraling unmet social needs, social isolation, and financial insecurity.

All this, of course, has profound effects on your own life as well as the patient's, even though to others it might seem that only the patient is going through major changes. All the attention seems to be focused on him/her. You may feel guilt, too, because of your own good health.

This combination, on top of your efforts to understand and help your loved one, can add up to a significant burden. You may neglect your own needs in your effort to take care of the FMS patient and the family, but it is important not to let this happen.

15

Remember:

**If you don't take care of yourself you
will be of no help to anyone else.**

Friends' and family's ability to cope with FMS is greatly influenced by the perception they have of the condition. The need for education can not be emphasized enough. Only knowledge and understanding will enable you or your loved one to make informed healthcare decisions and achieve a restored sense of order and control to your lives.

A sense of control is a key element in managing a medical condition. Its importance was emphasized in a course called The Arthritis Self-Help Course, for people with arthritis and fibromyalgia (added to the course in 1995)[5]. The six-week program, given two hours per week, teaches self management techniques.

Results from this study show that people who take this course increased their knowledge about their condition and developed healthier habits, such as exercise and relaxation, which resulted in a decrease of pain and depression. However, it was learned that the reason the course "worked" was not because of the changed behaviors, but rather because of people's beliefs about how much control they have over their pain. In other words, when people are confident that they have some control over their pain, the pain lessens. This also holds true for family and friends of the person with the medical condition. You can either feel influential or powerless over the situation depending on the information you have and how much control you feel over your own life.

Gaining knowledge is the key to gaining control.

One way to gain more control is to recognize the responses or stages of feelings and emotions you and the FMS patient will probably experience as you adjust to the condition.

Stages of Loss

The feelings and emotions experienced from the challenges of a painful medical condition are commonly expressed as stages of loss. For the patient, it may be the loss of an energetic lifestyle or it may be the loss of the ability to perform previously simple tasks such as sitting at a computer for more than 30 minutes at a time without pain. For you, it may be the loss of companionship in activities you use to share, or it may be the loss of having relaxed enjoyable conversations with your companion.

No matter how great or small the loss, several common stages of loss are recognized. If you're familiar with these stages, recognizing them will give you a greater understanding of the steps necessary in making changes.

The five responses commonly associated with loss are:
- Denial
- Anger
- Bargaining
- Depression
- Acceptance

These stages aren't always experienced in sequence. You and the FMS patient may move back and forth among them more than once. With any condition that waxes and wanes, there is often a need to recycle through the stages to some degree when confronted with a new painful episode. Recognizing where you or your loved one may be in these stages will usually help you to move through them more quickly.

Denial

Denial is very common in all chronic conditions. Initially, having a diagnosis at all may give the FMS patient a sense of relief, after months or even years of feeling like their pain wasn't real because tests don't show abnormalities. The validation of a diagnosis assures the patient that the pain isn't "all in their minds" after all. But a denial response may occur after their pain is validated. The patient will need and constantly look for reassurance about the reality of his/her condition from loved ones.

The patient's denial response may come in the form of statements such as "Oh no, this can not be happening to me." You may also experience feelings of denial. Many family members want to deny the painful nature of fibromyalgia and hold out hope that the condition is imaginary, that "only" psychological factors are involved. Sometimes this comes from a belief that the patient's condition will be resolved more easily if the symptoms are emotionally caused. Another, less open factor, can be the hope that if the patient's personal psychological factors are the only cause of the condition, then it may not be necessary to confront the issues of how the family will have to change and adapt.

Anger

A patient's feeling of anger will probably take some form of feelings or statements like "Why me? What did I do to deserve this?" You, too, may feel angry about the disruption of FMS in your life and feel the same things. Anger can also be your reaction to costly treatment that you don't agree with because it seems so "alternative," or ineffective. Feelings of anger are real and appropriate when you are faced with a disruption such as fibromyalgia. It's essential to find outlets for expressing anger if you are going to be able to maintain a caring relationship. You might want to consider finding someone you trust to listen to you and acknowledge your anger, either a close friend or a psychotherapist, or consider attending a support group meeting where others can understand and relate to your feelings.

Bargaining

Bargaining means trying to make the problem go away if only the patient tries to be a better person–however he/she interprets that. Often the patient starts looking for a quick fix, or launches an exhaustive search for the "right" doctor or therapy. Family members may try to bargain–to get things "back to normal"–by convincing themselves that if they're more patient or less critical then maybe the FMS will go away. This is particularly true with children. Children may say to themselves, "If I just clean my room or do all the things Mom or Dad tells me to do, maybe there won't be so much pain." Children are very vulnerable to disruptive changes in the family and need constant reinforcement that it is not their fault.

Depression

Depression's role in conditions like fibromyalgia has recently gotten more attention from the medical community. One is at risk for depression just by having a medical condition. Patients who see their health as poor are more likely to have severe depressive symptoms than patients who see their health as excellent. The more severe the pain, the greater the disability or the more unpredictable the condition, the greater the risk of depression. A condition that can wreak havoc on your life, employment, finances and relationships can foster that lack of control, which often spirals downward into depression.

Given what you now know about fibromyalgia, you will most likely understand that for the FMS patient, depression can be a very large part of coping with this condition. You, too, might also have depressive episodes because of the disruption in your life. It's important to be on the alert for signs of depression in the patient and yourself.

The risk factors for depression include: being a woman, prior depressive episodes, a medical condition, very little or no social support, a stressful life event, or family history of depressive disorders. This self-test from the Arthritis Foundation will help you see if you or the FMS patient should get treatment for depression:

A SELF TEST

Experiencing one or more of these depressive symptoms every now and then is a normal part of life. If a certain number of these have been bothering you for weeks or years, you may have a depressive disorder and should consult your doctor with this list in hand (see "Results" below).

GROUP 1: Are you experiencing at least one of the following nearly every day?

- Apathy, or loss of interest in things you used to enjoy, including sex
- Sadness, blues or irritability

GROUP 2: In addition, are you experiencing any of these?
- Feeling slowed down or restless
- Feeling worthless or guilty
- Changes in appetite or weight (a loss or gain of either)
- Thoughts of death or suicide (not necessarily attempts at suicide)*
- Problems concentrating, thinking, remembering or making decisions
- Trouble falling asleep or sleeping too much
- Loss of energy, feeling tired all the time

GROUP 3: And what about these symptoms? These are not used to diagnose depressive disorders, but often occur with them:
- Headaches**
- Other aches and pains**
- Digestive problems**
- Sexual problems**
- Feeling pessimistic or hopeless
- Being anxious or worried
- Low self-esteem

RESULTS

You may be in a major depressive episode if you are experiencing at least one of the symptoms in Group 1 and at least four of the symptoms in Group 2 nearly every day for at least two weeks.

You may have dysthymia, or chronic depression, if you are experiencing at least one of the symptoms in Group 1 and at least two of the symptoms in Group 2 nearly every day for at least two years.

* Suicide attempts or thoughts are never a part of healthy thought patterns and should never be written off as "the blues." If you have these thoughts, seek professional help.

** These are potential indications of depression only if not caused by another disease.

Depression feeds on depression; it's important to break the cycle. Focus on what you *can* accomplish. When you believe that things will get better, you increase the odds that they will.

Acceptance

Acceptance comes when you can acknowledge the adjustments you need to make and begin to learn effective coping mechanisms. An important part of acceptance is learning to communicate needs to one another. As a friend or family member, you can support the FMS patient by helping them discover new strengths and capabilities and by exploring pleasurable hobbies and activities–in short, by looking at what *can* still be done to enjoy life instead of what *cannot*.

Over/under participation

How you go about helping your loved one to better health has a significant impact on your own health and your loved one's health. How do you figure out how to participate?

A balance between caring for your own needs and being sensitive to the needs of the person you care about is best.

Overparticipation in the FMS patient's illness, in its extreme form, is doing everything for that person and not taking care of your own needs. People who overparticipate feel that their needs are not as important as the needs of their loved ones. The danger is that, if you don't share your own needs, the FMS patient can begin to feel even more helpless. There must be reciprocity, otherwise depression and isolation are likely to set in. Families who are too focused on the pain can unwittingly perpetuate it by encouraging it.

It's important to look closely at the support and nourishment you need in order to stay healthy yourself, and find ways to get them. It is critical to take charge of your own health. If your own energy is spent, then there is no energy left for your loved one either. Finding healthy outlets for releasing your own emotions can be a tremendous help in giving you the patience to cope with the needs of the FMS patient.

Underparticipation comes from not understanding fibromyalgia and finding it very uncomfortable to think about. You may feel irritated by hearing about symptoms, particularly pain. Or you may feel awkward and ill at ease when suffering and fear are expressed. Underparticipating in a loved one's problems can send a message of not caring.

Again, balance is the key. It takes courage to really listen to painful expressions of feelings and not make judgments or try to fix the problem. Close friends and family need to listen and risk being totally open to one another.

Effective Participation

A study of patients with rheumatoid arthritis, another chronically painful condition, gives valuable insights into ways of helping the FMS patient. When the arthritis patients were asked which things people said or did that helped them cope with their illness and which things only added further strain, the results were as follows:

Helpful gestures of support

- Giving the opportunity to express feelings and concerns.
- Offering encouragement, hope and optimism.
- Offering welcome advice and information.

Unhelpful gestures

- Minimizing severity of illness.
- Pessimistic comments.
- Expressing pity or overly solicitous attitudes.

The simplest and most direct approach to participating in the process is to let the FMS patient know that you care, to stay involved, and keep the lines of communication open by simply asking, "What can I do for you?"

Successful Families

There has been some research on families who have successfully adapted to the disruptive effects a chronic condition can have on the family–and by "family" we include the close friends that make up the patient's support system. It shows that families who successfully adjust or adapt to their situation not only consider the situation manageable but have, or can get, the necessary resources to meet the challenge. Once again, we are reminded of the importance of feeling in control of the situation.

Families that have been able to adapt have been defined as resilient–flexible, and able to recover from pressures. Traits of resilient families include:

- Successfully manage finances
- Communicate well
- Pursue leisure activities
- Have or build support networks
- Manage their time
- Establish routines

- Observe traditions

Resilient families also have a set of goals which are important factors in helping them cope with the challenges of chronic illness.

Family goals should provide for the biological, psychological and social development and maintenance of family members. Each member must be free to seek fulfillment of his/her individual needs, and feel they can achieve their own personal goals. When the family is confronted with an illness, members must not focus entirely on nurturing and protecting the patient (over-participation). It's important for each member to have personal autonomy and take part in social activities outside the family. When one member is diagnosed with a chronic illness, the family goals, and each family member's goals, need to be reevaluated with considerable thought given to new realities.

Making adjustments

Trust is the key to making family adjustments work. Many trust issues arise in the face of a disorder like FMS because it is *invisible.* The FMS patient needs to trust that the family validates his/her condition, and will be compassionate and understanding about the limitations the condition brings. The family, on the other hand, needs to trust the FMS patient to not always focus on the illness, or to need constant attention and care. The family needs to strive for hope and optimism, and also know that the patient will try to be hopeful and optimistic as well. Finally, the family and the FMS patient need quality companionship with each other.

People with FMS especially need to be trusted by those closest to them. It is very hard for both them and those around them to believe and trust without the real evidence of clinical findings. "I don't have as much pain today," or "I feel much worse this week" aren't as simple and convincing as "My white cell count is down," or "The X-rays showed less healing." If the patient doesn't feel trusted, he or she may feel a need to exaggerate symptoms in order to be believed. The need for validation is so great that it will be sought after until some acknowledgment is made.

We hope it is apparent from this discussion that the impact of fibromyalgia extends beyond the patient and into his/her closest and most precious relationships. We never know what challenges life will present us with or how well we will make those adjustments and adaptations. Because we are human beings existing in the world together, we have an impact on each others lives, sometimes a welcome one and sometimes unwelcome. Meeting the challenges of a crisis, such as a disruptive medical condition, can give you a great sense of accomplishment and satisfaction. It can lift you up rather than beat you down. A life crisis is truly an opportunity to find out what is really important to you.

IMPORTANT ASPECTS OF SUPPORT

You can help support the FMS patient in many ways. In listing some of them below, we don't want to imply that you or any one person should be giving support in all of these ways all of the time. These are simply some of the ways to show you care.

Education

Knowing about the condition is the only way to understand what the FMS patient is going through and how you can help the adjustment.

You are reading one source for information. In addition, today's world offers many ways to research FMS: through public libraries, the Internet and World Wide Web, and medical libraries or Infotrac (a computerized search of popular journals), to name just a few. Most of these are readily available. Even if you live in a remote area, you can write or call medical or information retrieval services in cities near you to see what they have to offer.

However, it is important to know that *the literature about fibromyalgia is very controversial and can be confusing.* You'll be less frustrated by your research if you keep this in mind from the start. To begin with, it is most helpful to get a basic understanding of the condition and some idea of the most effective treatment approaches. Beyond that, you can then explore other material that reflects current thinking and various philosophies on treating FMS. Remember to be careful about being misled by articles that are written negatively and hold out no hope for improvement. These are not only wrong–they can have a devastating effect on the healing process.

We live in an information society and there are many sources you can tap into. For example, the Arthritis Foundation is a national organization in Atlanta, Georgia which has many chapter offices around the country and can be a great source of help.[7] The Foundation offers many helpful and free patient educational brochures, including one specifically related to fibromyalgia. In addition, the Foundation might be able to refer you to a self-help course or a support/education group for FMS patients in your area. This can be helpful for both you and your friend or family member. Treatment and support groups can do much to relieve feelings of isolation, and gives both you and the FMS patient a safe, comfortable environment for sharing concerns and advice with others who understand what you're facing. A support/education group can also be a great way to find out about other resources within your community as well as how others are learning to live with fibromyalgia.

As you learn more about FMS and how other people cope with chronic conditions, you'll learn what kinds of situations are helpful and which are damaging.

Knowing that lightning is followed by thunder prepares you for the booming sound that follows the flash of light. Likewise, if you know that the FMS patient is made anxious by social situations involving many strangers, you can avoid those events or make sure he/she is accompanied by a friend. If you know that having a dinner party for friends or attending a family reunion is stressful for the FMS patient, then you can address and discuss that issue ahead of time and possibly avoid unnecessary pain. Becoming more aware of your reactions to certain events is an important way to learn about how you can better manage life's difficult situations.

Another way to gain more knowledge and understanding is to go along on one or more visits to his/her physician. You can ask questions of your own about things that might be puzzling you, or help the patient remember questions that came up earlier.

Physician Relationships

When we think of support for painful medical conditions, we often rely primarily on healthcare providers for that support. One of our hopes in writing this booklet is to help change that dependence on "experts" alone.

It is extremely important not to rely solely on the physician or any other health care provider for answers and support.

As discussed earlier, most physicians have not had much success in treating FMS. Many of the answers to questions about FMS are best–or only–found within the patient him/herself (the healer within). It is truly up to the patient and those closely involved with him/her to tap into all available resources and learn how to make the needed adjustments in the management of this condition.

To be sure, physicians and other healthcare providers have medical backgrounds. However, it's important to realize the limitations of their knowledge as well as its extent. Physicians and other healthcare providers have very specialized scientific knowledge. Most of them can offer expertise, knowledge and assistance with treatments involving drugs, surgery, physical therapy and other direct treatment approaches. But given the nature of FMS, with its lack of clinical findings, it is very difficult and frustrating for many physicians who try to treat it. Therefore, whether or not you have found a physician who understands FMS, the most effective treatment programs have been when the patient finds the supportive environment outside the physician's office, then uses the physician as a *collaborator* in designing treatment approaches.

Pleasurable Activities

Whether you are living with a disruptive medical condition or not it often seems hard to find ways to enjoy yourself. "I have no time" is too often the response to a suggestion of some outing or amusement. Our society moves at a fast pace. Monumental technological advances are around every corner, constantly challenging our ability to adapt. Competition is the theme; there seems to be an urgent need to produce, produce, produce, no matter what your role/job is, from full-time parent to corporate executive. Simple pleasurable activities are often seen as lazy and unproductive. Corporations reward those people who put in long hours and work on weekends to get the job done. Working parents who stretch themselves across work, school, childrens activities, health club workouts, and social activities are seen as successful and accomplished.

Unfortunately, we haven't figured out a way to acknowledge and reward a person for living a balanced life with time and space for quiet reflection. At times it seems as though our society might be starting to realize how short-sighted this is, as alternative work and life styles are developed. But so far it's still too true that simple pleasurable activities are under-valued in our culture.

How can we change this for ourselves? How do we break these habits that cause such great tension and stress, and which are so unhealthy for everyone? Is it possible that ignoring our need for relaxation and pleasure is part of what's causing the epidemics of chronic pain that our society is experiencing?

Pleasurable activities are best at their most simplistic level: appreciating a beautiful sunset or sunrise, inhaling the smell of cookies baking, getting a smile from your child, warming yourself at a blazing fire on a cold day, drinking a cool glass of water on a hot summer day. Small pleasures can help absorb some of the shocks and difficulties of life. Improving your health can also be viewed as a pleasurable experience.

It is our recommendation to make it a weekly goal to find and savor at least one pleasurable activity or moment. Then, once you're achieving that on a weekly basis, make it a daily goal. And if you are on a roll make it an hourly goal. Having FMS or any other chronic condition does *not* end the pursuit of pleasurable activities. Darlene Cohen, the author of *Arthritis - Stop Suffering, Start Moving*,[8] has been living with chronic rheumatoid arthritis for 18 years. She has adopted a phrase she lives by; "the relentless pursuit of pleasure!" Make this your most important life's work.

Power of Touch

Being touched is, in and of itself, a pleasurable experience–for both the giver and the receiver. To completely appreciate the pleasure of touch you have to be living in the moment and letting all your senses come alive. Touching someone with chronic pain can have a healing effect because it demonstrates caring. Touching with tenderness conveys affection and can be relaxing and very pleasurable. There's no better way to express affection or to comfort someone than to reach out and hug him/her. However, it's important that you learn how to touch someone with FMS. You must proceed slowly and with great sensitivity if someone is not used to being touched. The popularity of massage is a testament to how much people love the physical pleasure of being touched. Massage is a wonderful form of relaxation and gives everyone a way to enjoy being touched.

Optimism, Humor and Encouragement

Optimism, by its very definition, is the conviction that good will prevail over bad. That is not a bad thing to hope for no matter what our condition might be. Optimists will remember pleasurable events, look forward to pleasurable activities and downplay difficulties. For optimists, feelings of pleasure will last longer and positive moods will prevail over negative feelings. Do you see the glass as half empty or half full? Later, under "Coping Strategies," we will discuss in detail how to replace our negative habits with more positive habits, and show how this can help in coping with difficult life situations.

Being optimistic also means thinking about the things in your life right now that bring you happiness. We all have them. Some people have to dig deeper than others to find them, but they are there for everyone. When you're dealing with a person in chronic pain, it's important for you to encourage optimism in him/her as well as in yourself. Focus on how you have progressed in your life. How are you better off now than you were before? If you or your loved one find it impossible to find ways to focus on happiness, your past may have overwhelming unresolved feelings that need to be dealt with professionally.

One of the best ways to deal with depression is to look at life with an eye toward humor. Watching a funny movie has actually been shown to boost the immune system. When you laugh, your heart rate increases and your breathing is faster. Good, hearty laughter can also be very relaxing. Norman Cousins, author of several self-healing books, used laughter, by watching reruns of the television show Candid Camera and the slapstick comedy of the Marx Brothers movies, to help himself recover from a crippling arthritic condition. He claimed that ten minutes of belly laughter had an anesthetic effect and would give him hours of pain free sleep.

Being able to laugh at yourself can also help you stay healthy. Try to find the humor in tense and stressful situations. Life with FMS can be very serious at times, and by allowing yourself to see the humor in a stressful situation, you may be able to diffuse the threat of pain and divert the tension. People who like humor and use it in their lives are less likely to suffer distress when confronted with negative life events. A laugh can provide a face-saving way to express anxieties, fears and other difficult emotions to others. Finding ways to include humor in your life can improve its quality and ease pain.

We all have a great many talents and abilities. The more we tap into them, the healthier we become. As we find those abilities and realize that we are more than just a body, the less vulnerable we are to stress. Men and women who have many interests in life suffer fewer stress signs; most are less depressed and have fewer muscle aches. When you have a variety of interests, in trying times you're able to tap into different areas that can be fulfilling and a source of pleasure and positive feelings. This can help both you and your loved one through the pain with FMS.

Try to look at life optimistically, use humor to avoid taking life too seriously, cultivate diverse interests in your loved one and yourself–these simple measures can be the least expensive and most effective medicine anyone can prescribe.

COMMUNICATION

Good communication among family and friends is important for many reasons. It prevents misunderstandings, helps build support from family and friends, and clarifies our thinking. An open expression of feelings within a family is crucial to the overall health of its members. Because communication takes place between at least two people, learning good communications skills is helpful, not only for FMS patients, but also their friends and family. Improved communication can actually be a side benefit of coping with a condition such as FMS. Dealing with adversity can force you to focus on communication which, when it works well, brings family and friends closer together. Relationships are sometimes taken for granted, and facing a crisis together and learning to talk honestly about it can foster a more meaningful and cherished experience with one another.

Communication is the critical element in all healthy relationships; poor communication is the biggest factor in poor relationships. The goal in any communication is to feel like you have been understood. The harder people try to express their feelings clearly and completely to each other, the better their relationship.

True, it isn't always easy to express feelings. Is it worth the effort? Without a doubt, the answer is yes. When feelings are not expressed, those suppressed feelings allow problems to fester and will begin to create relationship difficulties. Maintaining a relationship over the long haul requires open expression of feelings so conflicts can be dealt with before they grow too big to handle at all. For an effective expression of feelings, you first need to be conscious of those feelings, and then be able to discuss them clearly and in a non-threatening way. We communicate with the world in many different ways. Communication can be verbal or non-verbal.

Verbal Communication

Let's take a look at verbal communication first. One very effective method of communication, referred to as "I" messages, has been used for many years. "I" messages are a non-intimidating way to express yourself. The opposite of "I" messages are "You" messages. When you want your ideas to be heard, they must be presented in a way so that the receiver of your thought is in the best frame of mind to hear what you are trying to say. Using "I" messages is one simple and effective way to do that.

- *"I" message*: "I feel frustrated. I don't think you're hearing me."
- *Countering "You" message*: "You never listen to what I say."
- *"I" message*: "I need some help carrying this firewood."
- *Countering "You" message*: "You should help me with this firewood because I hurt so much today."

Think about how you might receive hearing these different expressions. In these somewhat exaggerated examples, the connotations of the "I" messages vary greatly from the "You" messages. "I" messages are clear, concise thoughts which are factual and express only what the speaker is feeling or trying to do or say. On the other hand, "You" messages tend to attack the other person, which often results in a defensive reaction. The defense often closes the door to any further discussion or communication about the issue.

Using "I" messages is effective, because not only will it avoid defensive reactions, it also helps you to clarify how you really do feel or think about an issue before you begin to discuss it. If you have to begin a message with how you feel, you are bound to think about it more carefully before speaking. Here are some examples of ways to begin a sentence, or even a thought, using an "I" message:

- I hear..
- I see...
- I imagine...
- I expect...
- I interpret that to mean...
- I want to run away.
- I want to speak up.
- I want to do my part.
- I feel relieved.
- I feel worried.

- I feel confident.

From these examples you can see how important it is to speak for *yourself*. They show how we can take responsibility for and acknowledge ownership of our own thoughts, opinions, observations and feelings. To illustrate this point more clearly, consider some common words and phrases that avoid taking ownership: "Some people," "It," "Everyone," "This article said," "I heard." Using these generic words and phrases confuses the source of the thought or feeling and who owns the message. Personal statements expressed as "I" messages, on the other hand, will reveal who you are and will increase the personal quality of any relationship.

Another way to help clarify your feelings is to describe them. There are three ways of doing this:

1) *By name*: "I feel sad."
2) *By action*: "I feel like crying."
3) *By figure of speech*: "I feel down in the dumps."

Using descriptions will help you when you're describing another person's behavior. In some of these cases, using a "You" message might be the best way to make your point. However, it's important to do this with clear factual statements and not with evaluation or interpretation. Consider these statements:

Clear factual description: "You keep interrupting me."
Evaluation statement: "You are a self centered person. You never listen to ideas from anyone else."

Which would *you* rather hear?

When responding to someone who has made the effort to express their feelings, it's important not to deny those feelings. If someone says "I'm depressed," they don't want to hear "Cheer up." When someone says "I'm angry," acknowledge their feeling, don't negate it with an unhelpful response such as "Oh, just calm down." The implication in these kinds of negating responses is that it isn't okay to feel that way. It's much more helpful to explore these honest expressions of feelings. You may be surprised by what thoughts can be uncovered.

And finally, when you're confused about how your message is being received, get feedback on it. Verbal communication is positively within your control, but learning to use it well takes awareness and lots of practice.

Non-Verbal Communication And Helpful Listening

Non-verbal communication is done with body language, through facial expressions such as smiling, frowning, raising an eyebrow; through vocalization such as laughing, crying, sighing; through gestures such as shrugging and waving; through postures such as crossed arms or hunched shoulders. Non-verbal communication accounts for more than 75% of our total communication, so whether or not you're aware of it, you're communicating feelings to others even if you don't utter a word. The challenge is to be aware of what you are "saying" nonverbally and how your various body and facial expressions send messages. You want to make sure you are communicating with others in the way you really want to.

Most of us are much better at talking than we are at listening, and yet listening is probably the most important communication skill. Some people are innately good listeners. Most of us aren't, but the skill of listening can be learned and practiced.

Helpful listening and responding should reflect acceptance, respect, interest and a desire to help. It invites the other person to explore problems, clarify feelings, gain insights and make decisions. There are several levels involved in being a good listener:

1. Listen to the words and tone of voice, and observe body language. It is often difficult to discuss problems. A good listener will not only pay attention to the words, but observe how the person is speaking. What does the voice sound like? Is it shaky or confident? Is the speaker struggling to get an idea across (having trouble finding the right words)? What is the body language, tense or relaxed? If you pay attention to these signs, you can often find that more is being expressed than the words alone are saying. It's important not to intrude on another's thoughts and feelings aggressively, but sometimes gentle encouragement can start a productive discussion. Words of encouragement include:

- "Tell me more."
- "Oh."
- "Go on."
- "Yes."
- "Really?"
- "Sure."

2. Let the other person know you heard them. In each interview conducted for this booklet, every FMS patient said that one of the most helpful things friends and family had done for them was to simply let them know they had been heard and their thoughts and feelings were acknowledged.

3. Let the other person know you heard both the content and the feelings behind the problem. This is often referred to as "reflective listening," which means that you clarify what you believe the other person is feeling. When using this technique, it is critical to be non-judgmental if you want someone to open up to you. Helpful things to concentrate on and listen to are:

- Feeling words
- General content of the message
- Body language

4. Get more information if you need it. If you aren't clear about the feelings or the content of the message, it's important to get clarification. The simplest way to do this is by just asking:

- "Tell me more."
- "I'm not sure I understand."
- "I really want to understand, please go on."

Paraphrasing–restating the message in other words–is another way to make sure you've understood it. When you paraphrase what you thought you heard, focus on the content of the words rather than the emotions. Paraphrasing should be in the form of a question because people don't like to be told what they meant.

For example, assume Mary, who has FMS, says "I'm not sure I want to go to the dinner at your mother's house tonight. I don't know, she always cooks such fatty foods and she never has any comfortable chairs and I don't think she understands my fibromyalgia, either."

One possible paraphrased response: "Well, I guess you're telling me you don't want to go." However, with this response you're telling Mary how she feels, which may or may not be accurate. This could lead to hurt feelings and the end of the discussion. Another possible paraphrased response would be: "Are you saying that you want to stay home?" This response might lead to a more open discussion about how Mary feels about going out for evenings like this.

You may feel overwhelmed by the work involved in good communication. Expressing feelings and becoming a good listener takes awareness and practice. But, since you're reading this booklet, you're obviously interesting in working on some tough issues. Communicating effectively is an essential element in facing those issues.

Communicating Outside Close Relationships

So far we've been discussing good communication among the members of the FMS patient's family and friends. It's also important, when a medical condition is involved, to communicate clearly with physicians, employers and insurers. This can be very tricky for those dealing with FMS. Some common questions about communicating with others are:

- Whom should we tell?
- What do we say?
- When do we tell them?

37

- How much should we tell them?

Unfortunately there is no simple step-by-step procedure for communicating with people outside of your close network. FMS is often misunderstood, and you may get unhelpful advice or feedback when you talk about it with others. But it may be worth the effort and risk even so, if you can get one piece of helpful information or find a new understanding soul.

COPING STRATEGIES

A family's ability to cope with a disruption like FMS involves both the family as a unit and the individual coping skills of each family member. As we said earlier, to cope effectively, you must feel you have some control over the situation. But how much control do you have in a situation such as this, especially since you're not the patient yourself? How much help can you be?

Just as the FMS patient must believe that he/she has options in dealing with the condition, so must the family members and friends feel they have options in dealing with the disruptions the condition brings in their own lives. If you feel backed in a corner with no place to turn (no control), then you cannot cope effectively with any situation. What follows are some specific strategies to help you get and keep that crucial sense of control.

Positive Self-Talk

We've already discussed the importance of being optimistic and positive. But how can you keep a positive attitude while your loved one is in pain and your own life has been dramatically disrupted? Sometimes all it takes is a determination not to let this adversity get you down. If you firmly believe that you can handle anything, then you will be able to handle anything. One effective strategy for keeping yourself in control and able to handle anything is the concept of *positive self-talk*.

Everyone talks to him/herself either consciously or subconsciously; this is *self-talk*. It reflects–and helps form–the way we look at the world. Certain thoughts and things we say to ourselves lead to unpleasant emotions such as fear, depression and anger. Do you focus on the disability and negative changes in the FMS patient, or do you more often see the strength and positive changes in this person? Do you focus on living or worry about living? Do you see what does work or what doesn't work? If we can interrupt the negative or unpleasant thoughts–change the focus–and replace them with more positive thoughts then we are better able to cope successfully. *Positive self-talk*–verbalizing to yourself the positive things in your life–helps instill a positive view of the world. The opposite, of course, is negative self-talk–talking to yourself about only the losses and unwanted changes, which encourages an unpleasant view of the world. Try to become aware of how you focus your attention and what you say to yourself in different life situations.

In learning to cope with FMS, there is so much to be hopeful about! Many people have learned to manage the condition successfully and live active, full lives. It takes a great deal of effort, but it can be done. Positive self-talk statements like the following can be a big help in that effort:

- "I've met so many nice people as I learn to deal with FMS."
- "I've learned to slow down to a much healthier pace."
- "I'm learning so much about how to handle my own life through this process."
- "We'll take things one step at a time and I'm sure we can handle this."
- "My anxiety and fears are signals for me to relax."
- "Worry will only makes things worse."
- "I'm really learning to solve problems. I can tackle many new problems now."

These statements can be part of the ongoing story we tell ourselves, so when you tell yourself the story about what you are experiencing in life, make it a good one. And if you aren't happy with that story, rewrite it and take out the unpleasant parts.

Eliminating negative, pleasure-blocking stories is important for your health and happiness. During difficult times, many people kick into an automatic pessimistic mode which can get stronger and stronger until it takes command. If you sense you are being extremely pessimistic, ask yourself; "Am I blaming myself for something that's beyond my control?" Accepting blame is reasonable only when dealing with something you can reasonably be accused of having caused.

Another good question to help put your story into perspective is, "Am I expecting perfection in myself and others?" When you're confronted with a situation where emotions, fears and anxieties run high and are frustrated by your reaction to it, ask yourself, "How could I have handled the situation differently?" These are the internal thoughts and stories you must learn to be aware of and realize you can change. When someone you care about is diagnosed with FMS, accept only the part of the responsibility that is yours–to be there as a friend, listener and someone who cares.

Finding Healthy Outlets

It sounds simple, and it is: if your own mental health is good, you'll be better able to give support to the FMS patient.

Friendship networks are very important to family members of FMS patients. You might be able to say things to someone "outside" that you don't want to burden the patient or family with.

Another healthy way to vent your feelings is to keep a journal. When you find yourself cycling through feelings of frustration, anger or fear about a situation you may feel is out of your control, writing down those feelings in a simple stream of consciousness can relieve some of the anxiety and pressure. (It can also alert you to a negative story line you may have been telling yourself.) Many psychologists believe that writing down feelings is one of the most effective therapies for dealing with them.

It's helpful to keep a sense of perspective, to remember that life is dynamic and always changing, cycling through low points, then reaching new heights. It's also important not to lose sight of your own personal goals when coping with stressful situations. Balancing care for the needs of your loved one and care for your own needs at the same time is a delicate but important task. Learning the following problem-solving skills can help you meet the challenge.

Problem-Solving

Problem-solving skills are useful not only in coping with the challenges of FMS but in any situation that requires making adjustments and changes. Some common issues and questions that come up for families coping with fibromyalgia are:

- Inability to plan activities because of uncertainty about how the FMS patient will be feeling.
- A messy house because the patient doesn't have the energy to clean.
- Financial worries because of loss of job or disability issues.
- Who will do all the cooking?
- What kind of vacation can we take together?

Finding ways to problem-solve will help reduce the anxiety associated with these kinds of difficult decisions.

In the Arthritis Self-Help Course for arthritis and fibromyalgia, the following problem solving process is used. It may seem elementary if you happen to be the analytical type, but if you have trouble knowing where to start problems, this step-by-step process can help get you going.

1. Identify the problem: this is the most difficult step because you need to be as specific as possible.
2. Make a list of alternative ideas as to how you might solve this problem.
3. Choose the one or more that seems most appropriate to try right now.
4. Evaluate the results.
5. If not satisfied, then choose another idea from the list.
6. Check to make sure you are tapping into all of your resources.
7. Accept that the problem may not be solvable at this time.

The following scenario is an example of how this process can work:

Martha has recently been diagnosed with fibromyalgia. In retrospect, she relates the diagnosis to a major traumatic event in her life. Martha's mother, whom she was very close to, died suddenly one Christmas morning. Shortly after this event, Martha had debilitating muscle pain, sensations of numbness, tingling, dizziness and extreme depression. Until then, she and her husband, Joe, had led an extremely active lifestyle–running, hiking, bicycle riding, etc. Martha is an RN, and when her symptoms persisted, she began to worry that she had multiple sclerosis, so both she and Joe were initially relieved when the diagnosis was fibromyalgia although neither one of them know anything about it. Soon after she received this diagnosis she and Joe were out to dinner with a physician friend. The physician claimed that FMS was a "wastebasket" diagnosis. This has had a big impact on both Martha and Joe. Martha feels hurt and confused, and Joe is beginning to feel that FMS is a bogus diagnosis. Now Martha's symptoms are worse and she feels invalidated and hurt by her husband. Let's try using the problem-solving steps to help sort out some of these issues.

Step 1. *Identify the Problem*

Martha has a new diagnosis of a condition she and Joe know little about. Joe wonders if this diagnosis is just another way for the doctors to make money. He feels angry, confused, and resentful that his wife can't get the answers she needs to start feeling better. Martha knows her pain is real and feels abandoned and misunderstood by Joe.

Step 2. *List Ideas*

Ideas for Martha

- Educate herself about the condition by using research resources such as the Arthritis Foundation, libraries, and the World Wide Web for patient educational material.
- Call the Arthritis Foundation for information about education and support groups in the area.
- Ask her physician about all options for treatment and therapies.
- Use "I" messages to communicate with Joe about feelings and listen carefully to Joe's feelings.
- Practice positive statements about hope for the future and ways to enjoy life.
- Seek professional psychological help if unable to be positive and hopeful about the future.

Ideas for Joe

- Read the material about understanding FMS that Martha finds.
- Look for other resources (organizations, support groups) that might be helpful for himself as well as Martha.
- Accompany Martha on a visit to her physician to clarify unanswered questions he may have.
- Use "I" messages to communicate with Martha about feelings and listen carefully to Martha's feelings.
- Encourage Martha to list the activities that she is still

capable of doing.

- Find healthy outlets for stress and relaxation.

Step 3. Choose at least one idea each from the list to implement.

Martha and Joe should begin with the idea or ideas that they feel the most comfortable with, or that seem easiest to do. In this scenario, they both feel the need to get more information about FMS, so both decide to start by spending some time at the library researching the condition.

Step 4. Evaluate..

After Martha and Joe have pursued the library idea, they need to step back and assess whether or not they now have a better understanding of fibromyalgia.

Step 5. Choose another idea if not satisfied.

The library may or may not have been helpful for Martha and Joe. Often libraries will have no information or conflicting information on fibromyalgia. If this is the case, they need to refer back to the original list of ideas and try another one. It may be that they have to work their way through the whole list of ideas noted above to become more comfortable with the diagnosis and learn to communicate better with each other.

Step 6. Tap into all resources.

As they begin to do research and make contacts with organizations such as the Arthritis Foundation, Martha and Joe will probably find other untapped resources such as a support/education group or an FMS self-help course. Broadening a resource-base may be as simple as asking each contact; "Do you know of another source for information on this topic?"

Step 7. Accept that the problem may not be solvable now.

In this scenario, if Martha and Joe work through the entire

list of ideas, they should gain a better understanding of FMS, and their communication about feelings should improve. But not all problem-solving is successful the first time, so it's important for them not to give up. Just working through these steps together will help them learn how to approach problems, and should help lead to a better means of resolving problems in the future.

All of the steps in the process may seem burdensome at first, but it is important to go through them systematically the first few times. Then you can tailor the process to fit your own style, and much of it will become automatic.

Planning and Organizing

The first and most crucial skill in learning to plan and organize around FMS is *flexibility*. When you plan activities, have a back-up plan in case the first plan doesn't work out.

Flexible families do well in planning and organizing for the long haul of dealing with chronic conditions. Rigid families have a harder time, especially if the family is structured around traditional division of labor (Mom cooks, Dad mows lawn, etc.). Rigid families have trouble functioning when FMS breaks routines and certain things don't get done at certain times. These families need to find ways of doing things as more of a team. Around the house, it's important to find creative solutions so that all the essential jobs get done. First, determine which jobs absolutely must get done. Take a look at the chores that the FMS patient has traditionally been responsible for and try to divide them up or shift them around until he/she is up for doing them fully again. Then find ways to share part of that work. Giving everyone a voice and a chance to take part in the overall family goal will help create a sense of responsibility and teamwork. Sometimes just a little gesture–an offer to do a simple household chore or make dinner or take the family out to dinner–will take the pressure out of a difficult day.

It's important to plan for interesting and exciting activities or events in the future. But plan carefully, taking everyone's needs into consideration. There are many places to travel which can accommodate a relaxed vacation for the FMS patient and offer more active fun for others at the same time. It may take more creativity and inventive ideas to come up with solutions, but following the problem-solving steps above can help develop workable alternatives.

Taking a little extra time to organize your time and energy will go a long way toward helping your whole family adjust and adapt and find news ways to enjoy each other.

SPECIAL SITUATIONS

We have tried to write most of this booklet in terms that make it useful for both friends and family members of FMS patients. Now we want to focus on a few relationships and family situations that call for special attention, and offer a few thoughts and ideas for you to consider.

Partner/Spouse Issues

As the spouse or partner of an FMS patient, you're probably the most influential in coping with the condition as well as the most vulnerable to its stresses. First and foremost, you need to recognize how much your life has been affected by your partner's condition. It's hard to make necessary changes and confront important issues if you're not even aware of–or admitting to yourself–the need. Once you're in touch with how you have been affected, the next step is to identify the areas where you can help the situation. You must also recognize which elements are outside your control and therefore the responsibility of your partner.

One of the greatest challenges is to stay in emotional contact with your partner. Emotional contact is defined here as the ability to understand and express emotions easily. Remember that both of you need physical and intimate contact.

There are often intimacy problems during painful FMS episodes when your partner may have less desire for intimate contact due to a lack of energy or fear of more pain. Intimacy requires a full give and take from both partners. There are many ways to have comfortable intimate sexual contact with each other without pain, but finding them will once again require good honest communication between the two of you. During a painful period of FMS, some patients have said that simply lying close together was very soothing and comforting. Maintain physical contact in whatever way you can. It is, of course, a very individual matter between you and your partner how best to handle the painful periods and literally not lose touch, but it is so worth the effort. Intimacy and affection can be enormously important to healing.

We've already discussed how important reassurance, trust and validation are to FMS patients. As a partner, you're in the best position and have the best opportunities to give these. Remember that it's extremely important for you to validate that this condition is real and acknowledge the dramatic pain and sense of disability which often accompany it.

You can also reassure your partner by encouraging him/her to participate in the family in ways that he/she is still able to do. Ask your partner to take part in small ways at first. Success with small things will give you both a more solid foundation to build on, and let you progress to greater participation, up to the patient's comfortable limit. And when your partner does take charge, show your appreciation. This will go a long way to motivating him/her to continue to take on more responsibility which in turn will also improve his/her self-esteem.

But remember not to neglect the issue of your own self-esteem. So often your needs will be put on the back burner, particularly if there are young children to be cared for. But it's critical for you to set your own limits on how much you can do to help. There is no magic formula for doing this, but it may help to be aware of which of the chores or responsibilities you have taken on are making you feel resentment.

Feelings of resentment must not be allowed to build.

Some healthy partners may feel that they can't take care of their own needs because of all the additional responsibilities they are carrying. Practice saying no to activities that are not satisfying or that you resent every time you do them. You can't do everything and you should not try. If you feel resentful about doing certain things, you should take a long hard look at what you're trying to accomplish, and start to problem-solve with your partner to come up with alternative solutions.

When dealing with challenging partner issues, it can be helpful to look at what makes for happy everyday marriages. Some traits of successful couples are:

- Valuing each other
- Viewing the relationship as a unit
- Recognize relationship boundaries
- Communicate easily and clearly
- No power struggles
- Sharing a wide range of emotions
- Maintaining individualism
- Listening to each other
- Ability to negotiate conflict
- Sharing a value system

An excellent discussion of the importance of relationships in coping with conditions like FMS can be found in Maggie Strong's book, *Mainstay: For The Well Spouse Of The Chronically Ill.* If you work toward a solid foundation in your partnership, then the relationship should be able to withstand many earthquakes and still hold together.

Children Issues

If you are a parent of young children and your spouse has FMS, it's important to pay special attention to how the condition affects their lives. Ideally, raising children is handled with a delicate balance and equal participation by two healthy parents, so when one parent is "out of commission" that delicate balance is drastically altered. Your parental tasks, as the healthy parent, may increase until your partner begins to feel better.

Single parents with FMS are particularly in need of supportive, helpful friends. The parent should evaluate chores and tasks, decide which ones are essential for his/her family, which of these the parent him/herself must do, and which can be left up to others.

When fibromyalgia is part of your life the family must master two gears: 1) the "well gear" and 2) the "pain gear". Your children need to know which gear the family is working in at any given time, and what's required of them.

Young children must be assured that their own problems and needs are as important as anyone else's needs in the family, even if one member has FMS. Children will learn to sort out whose needs take precedent and are the high priority of the moment as they grow older, but only if their needs were met as children. Try to meet the immediate needs of a young child, even if the larger issues are out of control for a time. If parents can accept and incorporate FMS into their lives effectively, so will their children. As a parent, you are the ultimate role model for your children and being that role model is a never-ending job.

You, as a family, need to talk with your children about fibromyalgia. Young children have so much of the world to figure out, and they need so much from their parents. Many times parents want to shield their children from bad news to keep them innocent about the ways of the world. However, if you try to protect them from dramatic news, it will build a wall between you and them. Children sense when things are awry in the family whether they are told or not, so it is next to impossible to truly keep them innocent and unknowing. One way to incorporate your children into dealing positively with FMS is to involve them in the sharing of tasks. The more families share tasks and the more the parents are flexible about gender role division of labor, the better the children will feel about themselves. Helping out with family responsibilities is one of the best ways to build a child's self-esteem. And children can be a tremendous help, particularly for single-parent families.

A child may have both good and bad wishes about a parent. When a parent gets sick, the child may feel responsible because of those bad wishes. It is important to speak about life and the future with your children. Life will go on. Assure them that FMS isn't their fault. They may be afraid they'll have the same problems when they grow up. All these feelings and fears need to be expressed and addressed with children.

And last but not least, make sure you find ways to have fun. Once your children reach the age of mid-teens, if fun family activities have not been established, children won't be interested.

Stressful Times: Family Reunions, Holidays and Vacations

Because FMS can be exacerbated by stress, it's important to recognize potentially stressful times and figure out ways to minimize their impact ahead of time.

We all have our own unique relationships with our extended families. In all of the interviews involved in collecting material for this booklet, family relationships were singled out as being important–positively or negatively–in dealing with FMS. Our families confront us with a whole history of feelings and dynamics that all of us must find a way to handle, and this is particularly true for the FMS patient and you as part of his/her support system. Because most of us have to deal with our family whether we feel they understand us or not, it's worth the effort to try to develop some strategies.

There are many subtle–and not so subtle–emotions involved in dealing with family, that perhaps the first question to ask is, "How important is it to attend this family event?" Sometimes, you may be very close to your family and feel it is very important that you see them on a regular basis or attend family functions with them. But if your partner is having a hard time dealing with family get-togethers, it's important to weigh the benefits against the stress and FMS factors. Many times, while you attend the family function, your partner might prefer staying home, using the quiet time to rest and regenerate instead of attending a stressful event which may leave him/her exhausted .

If you skipped over the section on Communication, please go back and read it now (p31). When dealing with families, the emotions involved are usually very intense. Learning good communication skills will help you and your partner discuss how to be sure that both of your needs are met.

Holidays are particularly intense times. Our society places such an emphasis on holidays, it's impossible to ignore them even if you try, as you're bombarded with holiday messages on the radio, TV, shopping at stores, in your workplace, etc. However, in spite of all the commercial good cheer, holidays aren't always happy or festive times for people who are dealing with chronic conditions. Festivities take energy, throw off routines which may be important for health, may mean less rest, often involve eating and/or drinking to excess, and too often mean rushing around in a frenzy to get everything done. None of this is healthy for the FMS patient. Also, a disciplined approach to exercise and relaxation are two important elements of treating FMS; holidays aren't conducive to keeping to a disciplined routine for your health.

Extra understanding and support at these times is particularly important. Encourage your spouse to attend or be a part of

51

only those festivities that are comfortable and nourishing to his/her health.

A word about vacations and travel. Although many FMS patients may resist the notion of a getaway because of the effort it takes to plan one, or fears of being inadequate to the physical or psychological strain involved, a properly chosen and planned vacation may be the best thing for all of you. Try doing some problem-solving about where the fears lie and how they might be addressed. A change of scene can be enormously helpful in keeping FMS from becoming the sole focus of your lives

CONCLUSION

REMEMBER:

The pain of FMS is real.

FMS is a treatable condition.

FMS does not cause deformity.

It does not lead to arthritis.

It does not shorten life-expectancy.

If you understand, you can help.

If you don't take care of yourself,
you'll be of no help to anyone else.

Maintain your optimism and sense of humor. Learn and
practice coping strategies.

Communication is the critical element in all healthy
relationships.

Feelings of resentment must not be allowed to build.

Gaining knowledge is the key to gaining control.

It is extremely important not to rely solely on a physician or any
other healthcare provider for answers and support.

ABOUT THE AUTHORS

Betty Dotterer

Betty Dotterer founded and leads a support group for people who suffer from chronic pain problems, including fibromyalgia. She leads an Arthritis Self-Help Course for people with all forms of arthritis, as well as fibromyalgia. Betty currently serves as Vice-President of Programs for the North Bay Advisory Board of the Northern California Chapter of the Arthritis Foundation, and is involved in organizing and speaking on patient education information at public forums. She received a National Volunteer Service Citation from the Arthritis Foundation in 1996. Betty was diagnosed with rheumatoid arthritis in 1985 and resides in Novato, California with her husband and young daughter.

Paul Davidson, M.D.

Dr. Paul Davidson practices in Greenbrae, California and is a specialist in Internal Medicine and Rheumatology. He did his postgraduate rheumatology training at the Mayo Clinic, Rochester, Minnesota where he obtained his Masters Degree in Medicine, and at the University of California Medical School, San Francisco, California. He has long had an interest in rheumatology, and particularly in fibromyalgia and soft tissue rheumatism. He organized and is the Medical Director of the Fibromyalgia Clinic, Kentfield Rehabilitation Hospital, Kentfield, California. He has authored two books, *Are You Sure It's Arthritis?*, and *Chronic Muscle Pain Syndrome*, and has written articles for the medical as well as the lay literature. He has spoken extensively on fibromyalgia to both professional and lay groups, and has appeared on more than 100 radio and television shows.

REFERENCES

[1] Davidson, P., *Chronic Muscle Pain Syndrome*, Berkley Books, New York, 1989 and 1996.

[2] Wolfe F., Smythe HA, Yunus MB, et al: The American College of Rheumatology 1990 Criteria for the classification of fibromyalgia. Report of the multicenter criteria committee, *Arthritis & Rheum.*, 1990, 33:160-172.

[3] Froriep, R., *Ein Beitrag zur Pathologie und Therapie des Rheumatismus*, Weimar, 1843

[4] Gowers, W. R., Lumbago: Its Lessons and Analogues, *The British Medical Journal*, 1904, 117-121.

[5] Arthritis Foundation, *The Arthritis Self-Help Course*, Developed by Kate Lorig, R.N., Dr., P.H., revised 1995

[6] O'Koon, M., "Out of the Darkness," *Arthritis Today*, January/February 1996;34-40.

[7] Arthritis Foundation, 1314 Spring Street NW, Atlanta, Georgia, phone (800) 283-7800.

[8] Cohen, D., *Arthritis–Stop Suffering, Start Moving*, Walker Publishing Company, 1995

PROGRESS NOTES

PROGRESS NOTES

PROGRESS NOTES